Zouhour GASSARA
Hela FOURATI
Sofien BAKLOUTI

Ankle involvement in psoriatic arthritis

Zouhour GASSARA
Hela FOURATI
Sofien BAKLOUTI

Ankle involvement in psoriatic arthritis

Clinical and radiological aspects / Contribution of osteoarticular ultrasonography

ScienciaScripts

Imprint
Any brand names and product names mentioned in this book are subject to trademark, brand or patent protection and are trademarks or registered trademarks of their respective holders. The use of brand names, product names, common names, trade names, product descriptions etc. even without a particular marking in this work is in no way to be construed to mean that such names may be regarded as unrestricted in respect of trademark and brand protection legislation and could thus be used by anyone.

Cover image: www.ingimage.com

This book is a translation from the original published under ISBN 978-620-3-41375-5.

Publisher:
Sciencia Scripts
is a trademark of
Dodo Books Indian Ocean Ltd. and OmniScriptum S.R.L publishing group

120 High Road, East Finchley, London, N2 9ED, United Kingdom
Str. Armeneasca 28/1, office 1, Chisinau MD-2012, Republic of Moldova, Europe
Managing Directors: Ieva Konstantinova, Victoria Ursu
info@omniscriptum.com

Printed at: see last page
ISBN: 978-620-8-54638-0

ANKLE INVOLVEMENT PSORIATIC ARTHRITIS

CLINICAL AND RADIOLOGICAL ASPECTS / CONTRIBUTION

OF OSTEOARTICULAR ULTRASOUND

ZOUHOUR GASSARA HELA FOURATI

SOFIEN BAKLOUTI

TABLE OF CONTENTS

INTRODUCTION

Psoriatic arthritis (PsA) is a chronic, severe inflammatory rheumatic disease belonging to the spondyloarthritis family. Its prevalence is estimated at between 0.1% and 1% in the general population, and up to 30% in people with skin psoriasis. It affects men and women equally, mainly between the ages of 30 and 50 **[1]**.

Psoriasis is characterised by a heterogeneous and polymorphous clinical presentation combining peripheral joint manifestations (arthritis, synovitis, dactylitis, enthesitis) and/or axial manifestations (involvement of the spine and sacroiliac joints) as well as dermatological manifestations (psoriatic involvement of the skin and nails). Rheumatological manifestations usually develop within five to ten years of cutaneous psoriasis. However, 10% to 15% of patients develop joint involvement before skin involvement **[2,3]**.

involvement of the ankle (talocrural joint) is common Psoriatic arthritis, with prevalence ranging from 20% to 30% in the literature, it is often overlooked and unrecognised in patients with this condition **[4,5,6]**. In addition, it can be severe and lead to significant functional disability, thereby worsening the prognosis of this disease.

The objectives of our study were to :

1. To determine the prevalence ankle involvement in Psoriasis.

2. To study the clinical, radiographic and ultrasonographic characteristics of ankle damage in patients with RPso.

PATIENTS AND METHODS

1. Type of study

This is a cross-sectional, single-centre study conducted in the rheumatology department of the Hédi Chaker University Hospital in Sfax (Tunisia) over a period (June 2021-May 2022), including patients being monitored for RPso. Free and informed consent was obtained from all participants.

2. Study population

2.1. Inclusion

We included patients in our study:

- People with Psoriasis who meet the most recent classification criteria for Psoriasis (CASPAR) in 2006 **(Appendix 1),** regardless of how long the disease has been present.
- Aged 18 or over
- Who agreed to a clinical, podoscopic and ultrasound examination of the feet and ankles.

2.2. Non-inclusion criteria

We did not include patients in our study:

- Having another form of spondyloarthritis
- Carriers of congenital foot defects
- Foot or leg amputations
- Having refused clinical, podoscopic or ultrasound examination of the feet and ankles

3. Methods

3.1. Data collection

For all patients included, we collected:

3.1.1. Common data

- Demographic data: patient identity, age, gender, geographical origin, socio-economic level and profession.
- The patient's habits and personal history.
- The patient's family history: Particularly a history of skin psoriasis,

RPso or another form of spondyloarthritis.

3.1.2. Data relating to the disease

▪ **Clinical and radiological characteristics of the disease**duration of progression, age of onset, clinical presentation, clinico-radiological form (axial, peripheral or mixed), dermatological manifestations and other extra-articular manifestations...

▪ **Biological parameters**: inflammatory markers (ESR, CRP), HLA typing, rheumatoid factor (RF).

▪ **RPso evaluation scores :**

- To assess disease activity, we used the

ASDAS (Ankylosing Spondylitis Disease Activity Score) **(Appendix 2)**.

ASDAS is a validated score used assess activity and progression of the various forms of spondyloarthritis, including RPso **[7]**.

- To assess the functional impact of the disease, we used the **HAQ** (Health Assessment Questionnaire) **(Appendix 3)**.

HAQ is a functional score used to assess the impact of the disease on the patient's ability to carry out daily activities **[8]**.

3.2. Assessment of ankle damage

All patients included the study were screened and assessed for ankle involvement. Each patient received :

▪ **Careful questioning:** looking for functional signs pointing to ankle damage (inflammatory arthralgia of the ankle, joint swelling, etc.). If ankle pain was present, we specified how long it had been present, its intensity using the visual analogue scale (VAS pain) (0: no pain / 100: the most intense pain possible) and the time between onset of pain and the diagnosis of RPso.

▪ **A full physical examination:** including an examination of both ankles to look for pain and/or limitations to passive movement, synovitis, intra-articular effusion, etc.

All patients also underwent a podoscope examination to look for static disorders of the foot and a gait study.

▪ **Standard X-rays of the 2 ankles (front and side):** The standard X-rays were interpreted by the same rheumatologist experienced. The main radiological signs investigated were: pinching of the joint space, erosions and/or geodes and ankylosis.

▪ **An ultrasound scan of both ankles:** On the day inclusion and after the clinico-podoscopic assessment, an ultrasound scan of the ankles (in B mode and power Doppler mode) was performed by the same rheumatologist experienced osteoarticular ultrasound and blinded to the clinical data.We used an Esaote Mylab Gamma instrument with a line scan probe from 6 to 18 MHz.

The main ultrasound findings were synovitis, intra-articular effusion, cortical erosions and tenosynovitis. Tenosynovitis was detected in the fibular, posterior tibial, anterior tibial and extensor tendons of the toes.

4. Statistical analysis

The various data were entered and coded using IBM SPSS statistics20 software.After verification of normality by the Shapiro-Wilk test, the continuous variables were described in terms of means ± standard deviation. Qualitative variables were described in terms of percentages. For the analytical study, we divided our included patients into two groups:

- **Group 1:** patients with damage to the talocrural joint
- **Group 2**: Patients without talocrural joint damage).

Quantitative variables were compared between the two groups using Student's t-test and qualitative variables were compared between the two groups using Chi-square test ($\chi 2$). The significance threshold was a value of $\mathbf{p < 0.05}$.

RESULTS

The total number of patients followed up for RPso and included in our study was 40 patients.

1. Socio-demographic characteristics

1.1. Age

The mean age of patients was 49.9± 5.69 years, with a range from 22 to 80 years. The distribution of patients by age is summarised **in Figure 1**.

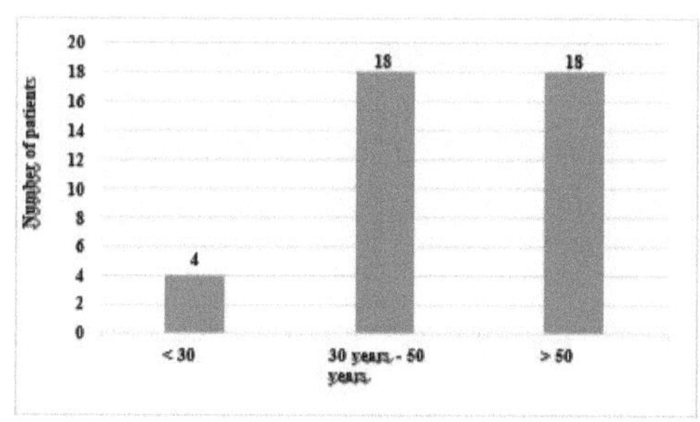

Figure 1: Breakdown of patients by age group.

1.2. Gender

There was a slight male predominance, with an M/F sex ratio of 1.2 (Figure 2).

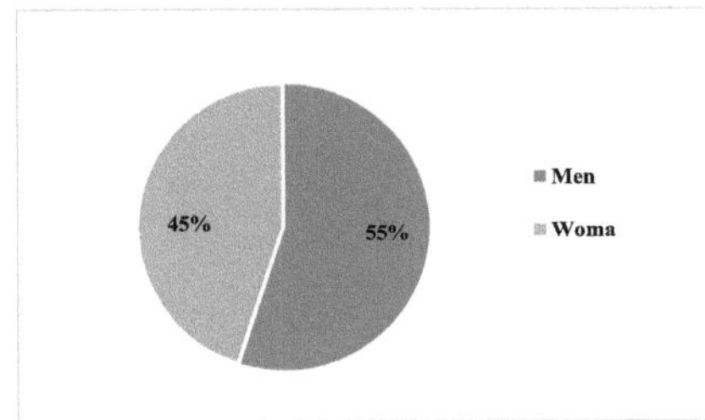

Figure 2: Breakdown of patients by sex.

1.3. Geographical origin

Seventy per cent of our patients (70%, n=28) were from central Tunisia and 30% of patients (n=12) were from southern Tunisia. Patients living in urban areas accounted for 62.5% of cases (n=25), while those of rural origin represented 37.5% of cases (n=15).

1.4. Profession

Thirty-five per cent of our patients (35%, n=14) were unemployed and attributed their unemployment to their illness-related disability **(Figure 3)**.

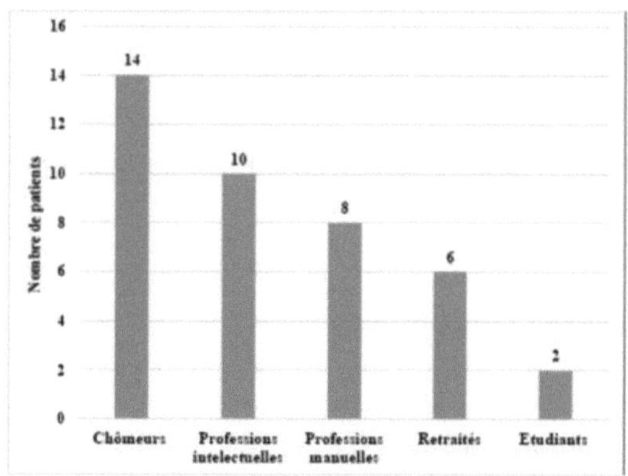

Figure 3: Breakdown of patients by profession.

2. Personal and family history

Smoking intoxication was reported in 27.5% of patients (n= 11). A medical history was reported in 52.5% of patients (n= 21), as shown in **Figure 3**. A family history of cutaneous psoriasis was mentioned in 15% of patients (n= 6) and a history of psoriatic arthritis in 5% of patients (n= 2).

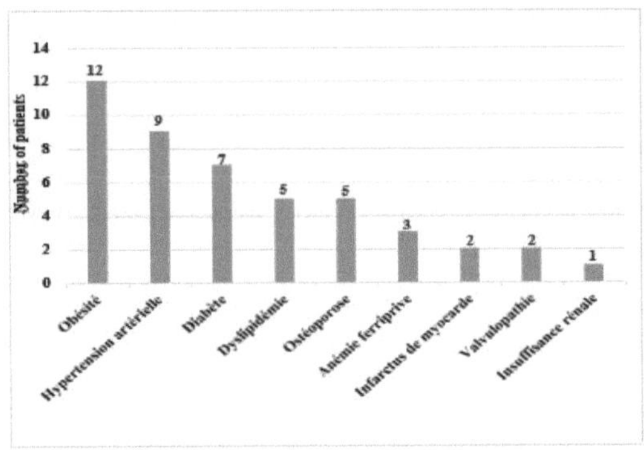

Figure 4: Medical history and comorbidities in our population.

3. Characteristics of the disease

3.1. Age at diagnosis of rheumatism

The mean age of patients at the time of diagnosis was 40.5 ± 5.45 years.

3.2. Development time

The average duration progression was 5 years, with extremes ranging from 1 month to 15 years.

3.3. Revealing clinical picture

The modes of onset were: oligoarthritis in 30% of cases (n=12), polyarthritis in 22.5% of cases (n=9), talalgia in 22.5% of cases (n=9), fessialgia in 20% of cases (n=8) and monoarthritis in 5% of cases (n=2).

3.4. Clinical-radiological form of rheumatological disease

The clinico-radiological form of RPso was pure peripheral in 52.5% of cases (n=21), axial and peripheral (mixed) in 42.5% (n=17) and pure axial in 5% (n=2) **(Figure 5)**.

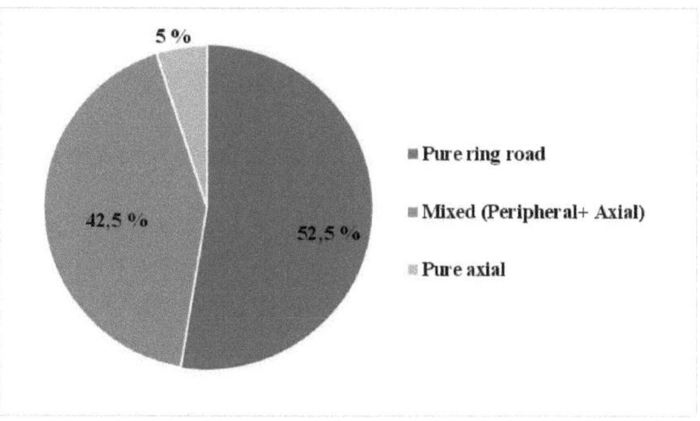

Figure 5: Clinico-radiological form of psoriatic arthritis in our population.

Clinically, peripheral joint involvement was found in 95 =The most frequently reported clinical symptoms were oligoarthritis of the lower limbs (35%, n=14), asymmetric polyarthritis of the hands (30%, n=12) and dactylitis (20%, n=8).Peripheral enthesitis was found in 80% of cases (n=32) and the heel was the enthesis affected in almost all of these patients (n=31). Axial manifestations (spinal pain and/or gluteal pain) were mentioned in 45% of cases (n=18). On standard radiographs of the pelvis: sacroiliitis was noted in 25% of cases (n = 10) (unilateral in 5 patients and bilateral in 5 patients) and coxitis was noted in 5% of patients (n = 2).

3.5. Extra-articular involvement

All our patients had skin and/or nail psoriasis lesions or a personal and/or family history of psoriasis. Psoriasis preceded rheumatoid arthritis in most patients (65.7% of cases), with a mean duration of 5.9 years before the onset of rheumatological manifestations. In 27.5% of patients, psoriasis was concomitant with rheumatism, and in 8.6% it developed after rheumatological manifestations. In addition to dermatological manifestations, extra-articular manifestations were noted in 12.5% of patients (n = 5): acute anterior uveitis (n = 3), IgA mesangial nephropathy (n = 1) and cardiac conduction disorders (n = 1).

3.6. Biological parameters

A biological inflammatory syndrome was noted in 62.5% of patients (n = 25). The mean SV value was 43.79 mm/h ± 29.14 mm/h and the mean CRP value was 20.83 mg/dL ± 28.06 mg/dL.The RF was negative in 85% of cases (n=34), slightly positive in 1 patient and not measured in 5 patients. HLA typing was performed in 50% of patients. HLA 27 was found 20% of these patients (n=4) and HLA B17 in 15% (n=3).

3.7. Disease assessment indicators

According to ASDAS activity score (VS), the disease was highly active in 67.5 % of cases (n= 27). The mean ASDAS score was 2.95± 1.88. With regard to the impact of the disease on our patients' quality of life, the mean value of the HAQ functional index was 0.9± 0.28 out of 3.

4. Characteristics of ankle involvement

4.1. Prevalence

In our series, ankle involvement was mentioned in 50% of patients (n= 20) **(Figure 6).**In these patients, the disease was symptomatic in 75% of cases (n = 15) and asymptomatic (discovered on imaging) in 25% of patients (n = 5). Ankle involvement revealed rheumatic disease in 25% of patients (n = 10).

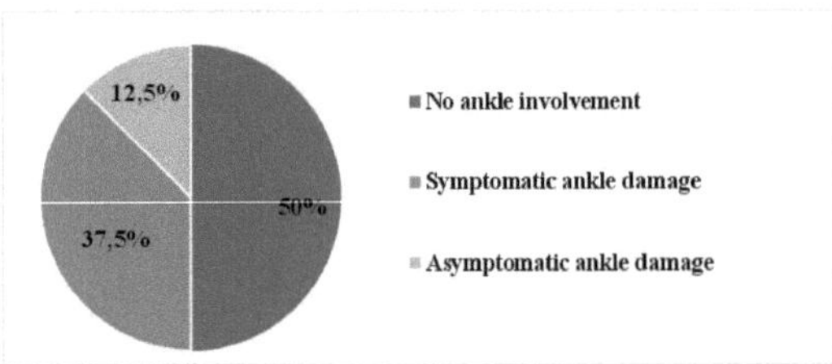

Figure 6: Prevalence ankle involvement in our population.

4.2. Clinical characteristics

4.2.1. Functional signs

Inflammatory arthralgia affecting one or both ankles was reported in 37.5% of our patients (n= 15). This arthralgia revealed the presence of Psoriasis in 25% of our patients (n = 10). The mean time between the onset of ankle pain and the onset of the disease was 6.7 months± 3.5 months, with extremes ranging from 0 to 36 months. mean ankle pain VAS was 58.25 ± 23.15.

4.2.2. Physical examination data

On examination, ankle arthritis was found in 30% of cases (n= 12). It was unilateral in 75% (n = 9) and bilateral in 25% (n = 3) of these patients. Other examination findings: Limited mobility of the talocrural joint (flexion and/or extension) was observed in 15% of cases (n = 6). Ankle instability was observed in 12.5% of cases (n = 5). Static disorders of the foot were identified on podoscopic examination in 27.5% of cases (n= 11): flat foot (n= 7), hollow foot (n= 1) and valgus of the hind foot (n= 3). Gait abnormalities were noted in 10% of cases (n = 4).

4.3. Standard X-rays

Standard ankle X-rays were normal in 70% of patients (n=28) and showed abnormalities in 30% (n=12). The radiological abnormalities observed were: pinching of the talocrural joint space (25%, n=10), erosions and/or geodes of the joint margins of the talocrural joint (20%, n=8), ankylosis of the talocrural joint (5%, n=2).

4.4. Ankle ultrasound

Ultrasound scans of both ankles showed abnormalities in 42.5% of patients (n = 17). In asymptomatic patients (pain-free ankle), ankle involvement was discovered on ultrasound in 4 patients. Of the patients with ultrasound damage to the ankle (n = 17), 47% had sub-radiological damage (no abnormalities on standard X-rays) (n = 8). Ultrasonographic abnormalities of the talocrural joint were: intra-articular effusion (27., n= 11), talocrural synovitis (15 %, n= 6), bone erosions (irregularities in the cortical bone) 12., n= 5) **(Figure 7)**. Ultrasonographic abnormalities of the ankle tendons (tenosynovitis) were observed in 30% of our patients (n=12). The tendons affected were, in decreasing order of frequency: fibular (17., n=7), anterior tibial (12.5%, n=5), posterior tibial (10%, n=4), Hallux longus (7.5%, n=3) **(Figure 8)**.

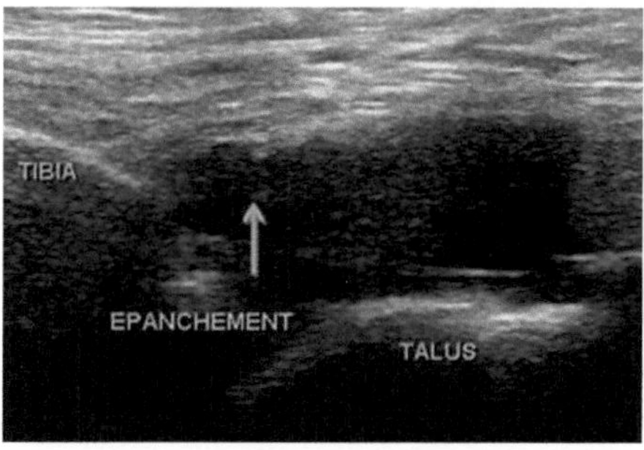

Figure 7: Ultrasound section showing talocrural arthritis intra-articular effusion

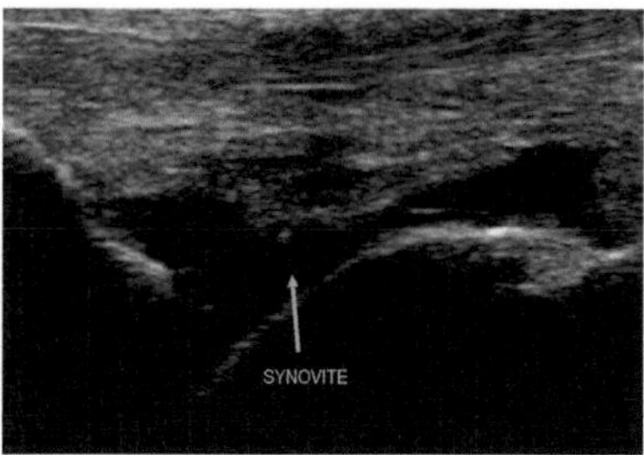

Figure 8: Ultrasound section showing talocrural synovitis

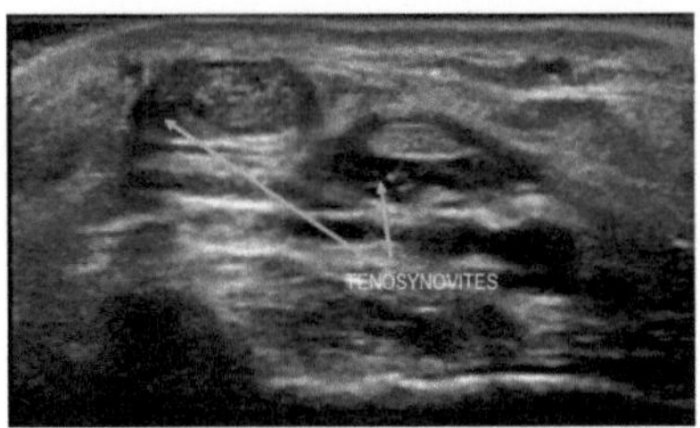

Figure 9: Ultrasound section showing tenosynovitis of the Tibial anterior and Hallux longus tendons.

5. Analytical study: Factors associated ankle injury

5.1. Socio-demographic characteristics

When comparing the two groups according to the presence or absence of talocrural damage, socio-demographic parameters did not appear to influence this damage in our study **(Table I).**

Table I: Comparison of sociodemographic parameters according to the presence or absence of talocrural damage.

	Group 1: Talocrural damage (+) N= 20	Group 2: Talocrural damage (-) N= 20	p
Age, years (average ± standard deviation)	51,8 ± 14,6	49,1 ± 13,8	0,55*
Sex ratio, M/F	12/8	11/9	0,89**
Unemployment, % (n)	40% (8)	30% (6)	0,39**
Smoking, % (n)	40% (8)	25% (5)	0,23**

* Student's t-test (quantitative variables), ** Chi-square test (qualitative variables)

5.2. Characteristics of the disease

A comparison of the two groups according to the presence or absence of ankle involvement showed no significant difference in body mass index (BMI), duration disease progression, presence of disorders of the ankle, or the presence or absence of ankle problems. statics of the feet or levels of biological markers of inflammation (VS and CRP) **(Table II)**.

Table II: Comparison of the clinical and biological characteristics of the disease according to the presence or absence of talocrural involvement.

	Group 1: Talocrural damage (+)N= 20	Group 2: Talocrural damage (-)N= 20	p
BMI, kg/m² (mean± standard deviation)	27.25± 3.11	25.54± 4.43	0,35*
Development time, months (mean ± standard deviation)	57.47± 38.25	48.16± 29.55	0,16*
Static foot disorders, % (n)	(5)	(6)	0,91**
VS, mm/h (mean± standard deviation)	47.71± 29.18	46.30± 23.92	0,88*
CRP,mg/L (mean ± standard deviation)	20.12± 12.51	18.90± 11.05	0,22*

BMI: Body Mass Index, SV: Sedimentation Rate, CRP: C-reactive protein

* Student's t-test (quantitative variables), ** Chi-square test (qualitative variables)

There was no significant difference in the ASDAS activity score (VS) between patients with and without ankle damage. However, a significant correlation was observed between the presence of talocrural damage and the HAQ functional score (p = 0.04) **(Table III)**.

Table III: Comparison disease assessment indices according to the presence or absence of talocrural involvement.

	Group 1: Talocrural damage (+)N= 20	Group 2: Talocrural damage (-)N= 20	p
ASDAS, (average ± standard deviation)	2,98 ± 1,2	2,92 ± 0,92	0,82
HAQ (mean± standard deviation)	1,12 ± 0,82	0,65 ± 0,32	0,04

ASDAS: Ankylosing Spondylitis Disease Activity Score, HAQ: Health Assessment Questionnaire.

DISCUSSION

Our study clearly demonstrated that ankle involvement (the talocrural joint) is frequent in subjects with Psoriasis. The prevalence of ankle involvement was 50%, and it revealed rheumatic disease in 25% of the patients included in the study. In the literature, the prevalence of ankle involvement varies between 20% and 30%, but it can be as high as 50% in some series, as demonstrated by our study **[4,5,6]**.

In all forms of spondyloarthritis, and more particularly in RPso, ankle involvement frequently occurs in the context of oligoarthritis of the lower limbs or polyarthritis, often asymmetric. Monoarticular involvement (monoarthritis of the ankle) is less common but may be observed, particularly in the early stages of the disease **[9, 10]**.

As with most rheumatic diseases, the main clinical manifestations of ankle involvement generally include inflammatory pain, abnormalities and difficulties in walking, arthritis, synovitis and tenosynovitis (particularly of the anterior ankle and fibular tendons). However, ankle involvement can sometimes be completely asymptomatic, and it is often imaging tests (particularly osteoarticular ultrasound) that enable it to be diagnosed, as in the case of 12.5% of our patients **[9, 10, 11]**.

In fact, ankle ultrasound is both reproducible and sensitive for detecting synovitis, intra-articular effusions in the talocrural joint and tenosynovitis, even in the absence of clinical signs. It can also reveal erosions and periosteal reconstructions not visible on standard radiographs, particularly at an early sub-radiological stage. In our study, of the patients presenting with ultrasound damage to the ankle (n= 17), 8 of them (47%) had no structural damage on standard X-rays. The first strong point of our study is the interest we have shown in ankle involvement during the course of RPso. Ankle involvement is often neglected, underestimated and insufficiently studied in this disease, even though it is frequently present. To the best of our knowledge, this is the first nationwide study on this subject. Another strength of our study is the global approach to talocrural joint involvement, which made it possible to study not only its clinical and radiological aspects, but also to include ultrasound exploration for all participants.In addition to the descriptive study, our work included a comparative analytical study between the two groups (according to the presence or absence of talocrural involvement) in order to study the factors associated with this involvement in our population. No significant associations were found between ankle involvement and other factors such as age, sex, BMI, duration disease progression, presence of static foot disorders, levels of biological markers of inflammation (VS and CRP) or ASDAS disease activity score. In the literature, there are no studies that have specifically evaluated the factors associated with ankle involvement in patients with Psoriasis. However, some studies have shown that men with Psoriasis are more likely to develop peripheral arthritis, regardless of location, than women, although these studies do not specify whether the ankles are specifically involved. This was not demonstrated in our series and no difference between the two sexes was observed **[12]**.

As far as BMI is concerned, there no published studies specifically looking at the association between ankle involvement and BMI during RPso. However, in other similar rheumatic diseases such as rheumatoid arthritis and polyarticular juvenile idiopathic arthritis, a significant association between BMI and the presence and progression of talocrural involvement has been demonstrated **[13,14]**. However, this relationship was not observed in our series, where BMI did not differ significantly between patients with and without talocrural involvement.In our study, the presence or absence talocrural involvement did not appear to influenced by levels of biological markers of inflammation or by the degree of disease activity (assessed by the ASDAS). Although, for example, the study by Yano et al **[13]** demonstrated a significant association between ankle involvement and disease activity according to the DAS 28 (Disease Activity Score) in the case of rheumatoid arthritis, there is a lack of studies on this subject in the context of osteoarthritis.However, a significant positive association was observed between ankle involvement and the HAQ quality of life score (p= 0.04), suggesting that ankle involvement contributes to worsening of functional disability and quality of life in these patients. In this context, it is well established that Psoriasis is a major cause functional disability due peripheral joint, axial and skin involvement **[15,16]**. According to the studies, the main factors associated with the extent of this disability in people with Psoriasis include the age of the disease, high activity and poor control of the disease, as well as the number of swollen joints **[17,18]**. Thus, the presence of arthritis is a determining factor functional disability PsORP, including ankle arthritis, because of the pain and walking difficulties it can cause. Our study had certain limitations and shortcomings, mainly the small sample size and the cross-sectional nature of the study, which did not allow us to follow the evolution of ankle damage over time. Further studies with larger populations and prolonged follow-up would seem interesting to obtain more reliable statistical results.

CONCLUSION

Our study demonstrated the high frequency of ankle involvement (talocrural joint) in subjects with rheumatoid arthritis, found in 50% of the patients included. In addition, it revealed rheumatic disease in 25% of the patients studied, underlining the importance of screening and assessing this joint in patients with rheumatoid arthritis. Our study also demonstrated the clinical and radiological polymorphism of this condition, with various aspects identified on standard X-rays and osteoarticular ultrasound.Ultrasound proved to be a fairly reproducible examination for assessing talocrural damage in our series, enabling the detection of synovitis, intra-articular effusions and tenosynovitis, even in the absence of clinical signs. It also enabled cortical erosions to be detected at an early, infra-radiological stage. Ultrasound should therefore become the main imaging test and an essential complement to the physical examination in everyday practice, to ensure better assessment and earlier detection of talocrural damage in patients with RPso. Another interesting finding of our study is that it showed a statistically significant association talocrural involvement and HAQ quality of life score in patients with Psoriasis, suggesting that talocrural involvement is a major source of functional disability in this condition, due to the pain and walking difficulties it can cause. Hence the importance of rigorous assessment of ankle involvement during the follow-up of patients with RPso, as well as early and appropriate management, in order to improve the prognosis of the disease and the quality of life of these patients.

REFERENCES

1. Karmacharya P, Chakradhar R, Ogdie A. The epidemiology of psoriatic arthritis: A literature review. Best Practice and Research: Clinical Rheumatology. June 2021; 35: 101692.

2. Choueiri M, Pina Vegas L, Claudepierre P. Psoriatic arthritis: diagnosis, criteria and boundaries. Revue du Rhumatisme Monographies. 2020; 87(4): 254-260.

3. Coates LC, Helliwell PS. Psoriatic arthritis: state of the art review. Clinical Medicine. 2017; 17(1): 65-70.

4. Tillett, W., et al. "Psoriatic arthritis: a review of the literature and management strategies." Clinical Rheumatology, 201; 30(4): 577-586.

5. Olivier, C. M., et al. "Prevalence and pattern of peripheral joint involvement in psoriatic arthritis: a study of 200 patients." Rheumatology International, 2008; 28(6): 547-550.

6. Rheumatology Department Study (2014). Study on the frequency of ankle involvement in psoriatic arthritis. European Journal of Rheumatology, 2014; 22(3): 175-180.

7. Van der et al. Sensitivity and discriminatory ability of the

Ankylosing Spondylitis Disease Activity Score in patients treated with etanercept or sulphasalazine in the ASÇEND trial. Rheumatology. Oct 1, 2012;51(10):1894-905.

8. Gudu T, Gossec L. Impact of psoriatic arthritis on quality of life. Revue du Rhumatisme Monographies. 1 Sept 2020 ;87(4) : 288-94.

9. McArdle A, Pennington S, FitzGerald O. Clinical Features of Psoriatic Arthritis: a Comprehensive Review of Unmet Clinical Needs. Clinical Reviews in Allergy and Immunology. Dec 2018; 55(3): 271-294.

10. Rida MA, Chandran V. Challenges in the clinical diagnosis of psoriatic arthritis. Clinical Immunology. May 2020; 214: 108390.

11. Galluzzo E, Lischi DM, Taglione E et al. Sonographic analysis of the ankle in patients with psoriatic arthritis. Scand Journal of Rheumatology. 2000; 29(1): 52-55.

12. Eder L, Thavaneswaran A, Chandran V, Gladman DD. Gender difference in disease expression, radiographic damage and disability among patients with psoriatic arthritis. Ann Rheum Dis 2013 ;72(4):578e82.

13. Yano k, Ikari k, Inoue E, Sakuma Y et al. Features of patients with rheumatoid arthritis whose debut joint is a foot or ankle joint: A 5,479-case study from the IORRA cohort. PLoS One. 2018;13(9):1-10.

14. **Bormann P, Ayhan F, Tuncay F, Sahin M et al.** Foot problems in a group of patients with rheumatoid arthritis: an unmet need for foot care. Open Rheumatol Journal. 2012 ; 6:290-5.

15. **Gladman DD, Antoni C, Mease P, Clegg DO, Nash P.** Psoriatic arthritis: epidemiology, clinical features, course, and outcome. Ann Rheum Dis 2005;64(Suppl 2):ii14-7.

16. **Kavanaugh A, Helliwell P, Ritchlin CT**. Psoriatic arthritis and burden of disease: patient perspectives from the population-based Multinational assessment of Psoriasis and Psoriatic Arthritis (MAPP) survey. Rheumatol Ther 2016; 3:91- 102.

17. **Mease P, Strand V, Gladman D.** Functional impairment measurement in psoriatic arthritis: Importance and challenges. Seminars in Arthritis and Rheumatism. 1 Dec 2018; 48(3):436-48.

18. **Haroon M, Gallagher P, FitzGerald O.** Diagnostic delay of more than 6 months contributes to poor radiographic and functional outcome in psoriatic arthritis. Ann Rheum Dis 2015; 74:1045-50.

APPENDICES

Appendix 1: 2006 CASPAR classification criteria for psoriatic arthritis

In the presence of inflammatory joint involvement (axial, peripheral or enthesitic), the diagnosis of psoriatic arthritis is made when **3 points are** present.

Psoriasis (one of the items) Current: 2 points Personal history: 1 point Family history: 1 point
2. Typical psoriatic nail : 1 point
3. Negative rheumatoid factor: 1 point
4. Current dactylitis or history of dactylitis diagnosed by a doctor :1 point
5. Radiological images juxta-articular ossifications on X-rays of the hands and/or feet (other than osteoarthritis): 1 point

Appendix 2: Ankylosing Spondylitis Disease Activity Score (ASDAS)

This is a score used to assess the activity of spondyloarthritis. It combines various parameters: overall spinal pain (0-100, question 2 of the BASDAI), morning stiffness (0-100, question 6 of the BASDAI), peripheral joint pain (0-100, question 3 of the BASDAI), patient assessment of disease activity (0-100) and CRP or VS depending on the formula chosen.

ASDAS disease activity thresholds

Inactive (Remission)	ASDAS< 1.3
Moderate	1.3≤ ASDAS< 2.1
Assets	2.1≤ ASDAS< 3.5
Very active	3.5≤ ASDAS

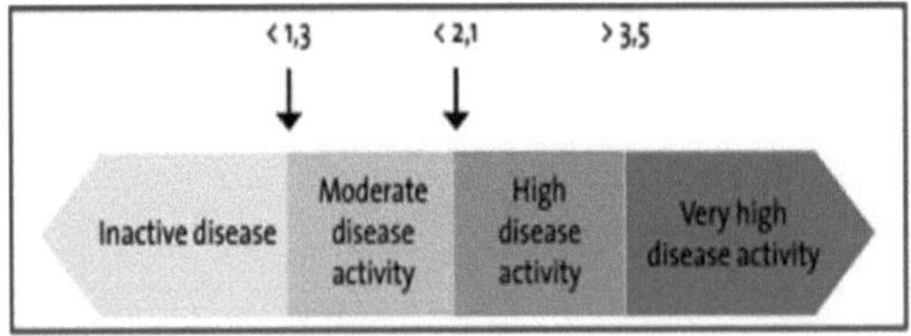

Appendix 3: Health Assessment Questionnaire (HAQ)

It is a functional score that reflects the functional capacity of patients by assessing their ability to carry out the activities of daily living in 8 different areas:

- Clothing and body care
- Getting up (from a chair, from bed...)
- Meals
- Walking
- Hygiene (washing, drying, etc.)
- Grabbing (lifting an object, picking something up off the ground...)
- Grip
- Other activities

The patient fills in the questionnaire. Each question is rated from 0 to 3 according to the difficulty experienced by the patient: 0: no difficulty, 1: some difficulty, 2: a lot of difficulty, 3: unable to perform the gesture.The score for each of the 8 areas is the score obtained among the answers to the questions in that area.The notion assistance from a third and/or the use of equipment changes the score to at least 2. A score of 3 is awarded if the previous score is already equal to 3.The HAQ index is the sum of the scores for the different areas, divided by 8.

HAQ between 0 (no disability) and 3 (total disability)

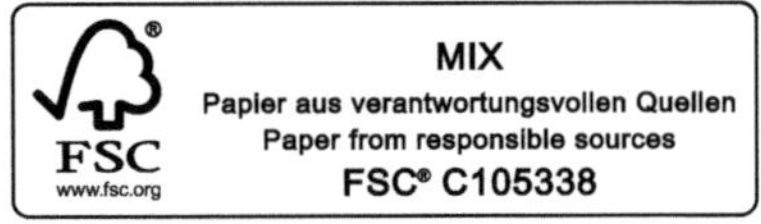

Printed by Books on Demand GmbH, Norderstedt / Germany